Mind's Gamble

Betting on the Psychology of Decision Making

Freudian Trips

Copyright Page

Disclaimer

The views and opinions expressed in this book are those of the author(s) and do not necessarily reflect the official policy or position of any other agency, organization, employer, or company. The contents of this book are for informational and educational purposes only and are not intended to serve as professional advice, diagnosis, or treatment.

The information provided in this book is believed to be accurate and reliable as of the date of publication. However, it may include some errors or inaccuracies, and no warranty or guarantee is provided regarding the accuracy, timeliness, or applicability of the content.

Readers are encouraged to consult with professional philosophers, educators, or other qualified professionals where appropriate for personalized advice. The author(s) and publisher shall not be liable for any loss, damage, or harm caused or alleged to be caused, directly or indirectly, by the information or ideas contained, suggested, or referenced in this book.

By reading this book, the reader acknowledges and agrees that they are solely responsible for how they interpret and apply the information contained herein.

This book may also include references to other works, studies, and sources. These references are provided for further reading and exploration and do not imply endorsement or validation of the specific theories, viewpoints, or interpretations presented in those works.

Chapter 1: "All In": An Introduction to Decision Making

As the sun's first rays crept over the horizon, Jenny found herself standing at a crossroad. Two paths lay before her. One was the familiar route to her usual morning jog spot, and the other, a new trail she'd never tried before. It seemed like a simple choice, but even here, in the quiet hours of dawn, she was making a decision.

Isn't life just a series of these? From the moment we wake up — deciding to hit the snooze button or jump out of bed, to the more significant life choices like career moves, relationships, and investments — we're constantly making decisions. Like Jenny, every day, we stand at crossroads, both big and small.

Every Day, Every Moment: The Story of Decisions

If you think about it, our days are filled with decisions. What to eat for breakfast? Which route to take to work? Should we even go to work or call in sick? Some of these choices may feel trivial, but they shape our daily experiences. Others, like whom to marry or what career to pursue, have long-lasting impacts on our lives.

Now, you might wonder, "Why should I think about decision-making? I've been making choices all my life without giving it a second thought!" That's true. But have you ever paused and pondered: Why did I make that choice? What influenced me? Did I make the right call?

Life's Big Canvas

Imagine your life as a vast canvas, every brush stroke a choice you make. Some strokes are bold and vivid, depicting major life events. Others are subtle, forming the background. But together, they shape the masterpiece of your life's journey.

Every decision, whether big or small, contributes to this grand picture. Sometimes, we're proud of our choices, feeling like the master artists of our destiny. At other times, we may wish we'd chosen differently. Yet, every decision offers a lesson, a new shade or color to our ever-evolving canvas.

The Unseen Forces at Play

Many times, our decisions aren't solely ours. Think about it. When you choose a vacation spot, is it purely based on your own desires? Or do friends' experiences, Instagram posts, or even the latest travel deals play a part?

External influences, past experiences, emotions, and even our innate instincts shape our decisions. Recognizing these factors doesn't diminish the value of our choices. Instead, it gives us a clearer picture, a deeper understanding of the 'why' behind our actions.

So, Why Does It Matter?

Understanding our decision-making process allows us to make more informed, confident choices. When we grasp the forces that sway us, we can steer our decisions towards what truly aligns with our desires, needs, and values.

Moreover, by recognizing that every day is full of these choices, we embrace the power and responsibility of shaping our destinies. No longer do we need to feel adrift in the current of life, merely reacting to what comes our way. We can become captains, charting our course with intention and purpose.

As Jenny took a deep breath and stepped onto the new trail, she embraced the beauty of uncertainty. She had made a choice, a decision, one of the many that would shape her day.

As you turn the pages of this book, embark on a journey to uncover the fascinating world of decisions. By the end, you'll not only have a clearer understanding of why you choose what you do but also be equipped to make choices that truly resonate with who you are.

So, are you ready to dive "All In"? Let's explore the intricate and beautiful maze of decision-making together.

Chapter 2: "Dealer's Hand": The Biological Basis of Decision Making

Imagine, if you will, the bustling activity within a grand casino. Amid the whirlwind of sounds, from the clinking of coins to the soft murmur of hushed conversations, stands the dealer. This dealer, with every card they hand out, dictates the game's flow, influencing players' choices and ultimately, the outcome of the game.

Similarly, within the casino of our minds, there's a 'dealer' guiding our decisions. This dealer isn't a person, but a complex network of cells, structures, and chemicals, all housed within our brain. Let's embark on an exciting journey to meet this dealer and understand how it influences our every move.

The Brain: Our Personal Dealer

When you think about making a decision, you might imagine it as a conscious, thoughtful process. But did you know that a large portion of this process is managed by your brain without you even being aware of it?

Imagine you're walking by a bakery. The smell of freshly baked bread wafts out. Almost immediately, your stomach rumbles, and you find yourself drawn inside. That irresistible urge? It's your brain at work, connecting the pleasant smell to memories of delicious, comforting food.

The Brain's Command Center: The Prefrontal Cortex

If our brain is a casino, then the prefrontal cortex is the VIP section. Located right behind your forehead, this area helps us make rational decisions. When faced with a choice, it weighs the pros and cons, considers past experiences, and predicts possible outcomes.

Think of the time you debated having that extra slice of cake. The voice urging restraint, reminding you of your health goals? That's the prefrontal cortex doing its thing.

Feeling Over Thinking: The Amygdala's Role

While the prefrontal cortex is all about logic, another part of our brain, the amygdala, deals with emotions. It's like that friend who insists you trust your gut feeling or follow your heart.

For instance, ever felt butterflies in your stomach before making a big decision? Or experienced a sudden rush of happiness when deciding to spend time with loved ones? The amygdala plays a crucial role in these emotion-driven decisions.

Chemicals in Command: The Role of Neurotransmitters

In our casino analogy, think of neurotransmitters as the chips. They facilitate the 'transactions' of information within the brain. These chemicals can influence our mood, feelings, and yes, our decisions.

Dopamine, for example, gives us a feeling of pleasure. When you're deciding between a salad and a chocolate dessert, dopamine might nudge you towards the latter because it remembers the joy of the last time you indulged.

Just as every card dealt in a game can change its outcome, various parts of our brain and the chemicals within it play a significant role in shaping our decisions. Recognizing and understanding this intricate 'dealer' can help us better grasp why we make the choices we do.

In the next chapter, we'll delve deeper into how these decisions evolve as we journey from childhood to old age. But for now, take a moment to appreciate the wondrous casino of your mind and the dealer that's always at play, guiding your every move.

Chapter 3: "Aces High": Decision Making Across the Life Span

Imagine a deck of cards, each one representing a stage of our lives. From the youthful exuberance of the Jack to the wisdom of the King and Queen, our lives are a continuous shuffle and deal of experiences. But have you ever stopped to think about how our decision-making evolves as we traverse through the deck of life?

Let's embark on a journey from the first card to the last, discovering how our decisions change as we grow older.

The Early Years: "Following the Leader"

The 2s to 10s of our deck

When we're young, our world is new and exciting, but also quite vast and complex. Think back to a time when you were a child, eager to explore but often looking up to the adults for guidance.

Children, in their formative years, primarily make decisions based on the world they're introduced to. It's a game of "Follow the Leader."

They rely on parents, teachers, and guardians to navigate them. Here, the choices are simple: which toy to play with, which story to read before bedtime. Yet, even these decisions are influenced by the safe environment curated for them.

The Teenage Years: "Testing the Waters"

The Jacks and Queens in training

Teenagers are like sailors in rough seas, navigating their ships through the tempest of hormones, peer pressure, and the looming responsibilities of adulthood. It's a time of rebellion, experimentation, and identity formation.

Their decisions are often driven by a mix of curiosity and a desire for autonomy. Remember the first time you decided to break a rule just to see what would happen? Or when you picked a hobby or interest that was entirely different from what your family expected? These are the formative choices that carve out our personalities.

The Adulthood Phase: "Playing the Hand You're Dealt"

The Kings and Queens of our deck

As adults, decisions become multifaceted. We juggle careers, relationships, finances, and personal growth. The deck is vast, and every card we play affects the game's outcome.

Here, past experiences play a significant role. The wisdom and lessons from earlier years shape our decisions. Think about the major decisions you've made — like buying a house, choosing a partner, or even selecting a job. Often, these are calculated moves, based on careful evaluation and long-term goals.

The Golden Years: "Playing with a Full Deck"

The Aces of our lives

In the later stages of life, people often reflect more than they project. Decisions become less about ambition and more about contentment, legacy, and understanding.

The pace might be slower, but each choice carries the weight of wisdom and experience. It's about cherishing memories, making peace with past decisions, and guiding the younger generation.

Just as in a game of cards, where every round is different, our approach to decision-making evolves as we progress through life. From the tentative choices of childhood to the confident decisions of adulthood, and finally, to the reflective choices of our golden years, our life's deck is always shuffling and dealing new experiences.

As we close this chapter, remember that no matter where you are in your life's game, every decision, every card you play, is a step towards understanding yourself better and shaping your destiny.

Chapter 4: "The House Edge": Rational Choice Theory

Imagine you're in a vibrant casino. The slot machines are chiming, people are placing their bets, and the roulette wheel is spinning. Now, let's say you're given a choice: bet on a game of pure luck or a game where you have some knowledge that might give you an edge. Which would you pick?

Most would lean towards the game where they have an advantage or some inside knowledge. This, in essence, is what the Rational Choice Theory is all about. It's like playing with the house edge, where you try to maximize your chances of winning by making the most informed decision.

Decisions at a Crossroad

At the heart of Rational Choice Theory is a simple idea: When faced with options, individuals will choose the one they believe offers the most benefit, while costing them the least.

Think about the last time you went shopping. You might have compared two similar products, weighing the pros and cons of each. Quality, price, brand reputation - all these factors played a role in your final decision. You opted for the one that promised the most value for your money.

All About the Pros and Cons

Just like when you're weighing the odds in a casino game, life often presents decisions where we must evaluate the potential gains against the potential losses.

For instance, imagine deciding between taking a safe, well-paying job or starting your own business. The job offers stability but perhaps less personal fulfillment. The business might promise independence and greater satisfaction, but with the risks of financial instability.

Through the lens of Rational Choice Theory, the decision would hinge on which option aligns best with your personal values, risk tolerance, and long-term goals.

But is it Always Rational?

While Rational Choice Theory offers a compelling framework, it doesn't mean we always make choices purely based on logical assessments. Emotions, habits, societal influences – they all can sway our decisions.

Yet, even these factors can be understood in terms of rational choice. For example, someone might make a decision based on societal expectations because they believe it will lead to greater social acceptance or avoid potential conflict, which in turn they value.

Applying the "House Edge" in Daily Life

Understanding the Rational Choice Theory isn't just an academic exercise. By recognizing how we evaluate choices and make decisions, we can become better, more informed decision-makers.

Next time you're at a crossroads, think about the "house edge." What do you stand to gain? What might you lose? And remember, the most rational choice isn't always about immediate rewards. Sometimes, playing the long game – thinking about future benefits – can lead to the biggest wins.

Life, in many ways, is like that bustling casino. Choices abound, and with each decision, we aim to maximize our gains and minimize our losses. By understanding and applying the principles of Rational Choice Theory, we can better navigate the game of life, always seeking that ever-elusive edge that tilts the odds in our favor.

Chapter 5: "Bluffing": Heuristics and Biases

Picture this: You're in the middle of an intense card game, and you notice a player consistently scratching their nose every time they're about to make a big move. Is it a tell? Or just a coincidence? Instead of analyzing each hand and calculating probabilities, you decide to trust this observation and make your move based on that.

This reliance on a pattern, or shortcut, is similar to something our minds often do, known as heuristics. But sometimes, just like in our card game, these shortcuts can lead us astray. Enter biases.

Mental Shortcuts: Why We Use Them

Imagine if, for every decision you made, you stopped to analyze all possible outcomes. From deciding what to eat for breakfast to which route to take to work, life would be an endless loop of analysis paralysis!

To streamline this, our brains use heuristics, or mental shortcuts. These help us make quick decisions without delving deep into exhaustive analysis.

For example, if a product is more expensive, we might assume it's of better quality, even if that's not always the case. This is a shortcut – it saves time, but it's not always accurate.

When Shortcuts Lead Us Astray: Biases

These heuristics, while handy, can sometimes lead to biases – essentially mistakes in our decision-making.

Let's return to our card game example. If you bank on that player's nose scratch as a tell, and they end up winning big, you've fallen for a bias. You relied too heavily on a mental shortcut without considering all the evidence.

There are numerous ways biases show up in our lives:

Confirmation Bias: We favor information that confirms our existing beliefs. For example, if we believe that a particular brand is the best, we might only notice reviews that praise it and ignore critical ones.

Overconfidence Bias: We believe in our own abilities too much. Think of a time when you were sure your team would win, only to be surprised by the outcome.

Stereotyping: This is a big one. We might make assumptions about someone based on their appearance, age, or background, without truly understanding them.

Guarding Against the Bluff

So, how do we ensure we're not being duped by our own minds?

Awareness: Simply knowing that these heuristics and biases exist is the first step. Once you're aware, you can catch yourself in the act.

Slow Down: Not every decision needs to be lightning fast. For important choices, take a moment to reflect. Are you relying on a shortcut, or have you considered all angles?

Seek Feedback: Two heads are often better than one. Discussing decisions with friends or colleagues can provide a fresh perspective and point out biases you might have missed.

While our brains are remarkable machines, they sometimes take shortcuts that don't serve us well. By understanding heuristics and biases, we can strive to make decisions that are more informed, more balanced, and less influenced by the "bluffs" our minds occasionally throw our way.

In our next chapter, we'll explore the social influences that shape our decisions, because as it turns out, we're not playing this game of life solo. Our choices are often influenced, in subtle and profound ways, by the players around us.

Chapter 6: "Fold or Call": Prospect Theory

Imagine you're at a high-stakes poker game. The pot is growing, and you've got a decent hand. Do you go all in, or do you play it safe? Sometimes, it's not just about the cards in front of you; it's about how you feel about those cards. This feeling, this emotional relationship with risk and reward, is at the heart of the Prospect Theory.

Let's dive into this intriguing world where our emotions, perceptions, and decisions intertwine.

The Game of Gains and Losses

Life, in many ways, is a series of gambles. Every decision carries potential gains and losses. But here's the twist: we don't always see gains and losses in the same light.

Consider this: Would you prefer a guaranteed $50, or a 50-50 chance of winning $100 or nothing? Many people would go for the sure $50, even though the expected value in both cases is the same. It feels good to win, and it feels terrible to lose.

Feeling the Weight of Loss

Prospect Theory suggests that losses hit us harder emotionally than equivalent gains. If you've ever been more upset about losing $20 than you were happy about finding the same amount, you've experienced this firsthand.

In the poker scenario, imagine you're on a winning streak. Would you risk your winnings? Now, consider the opposite - you've been on a losing streak. Do you chase your losses, trying to break even? This change in behavior, based on our emotional response to gains and losses, is central to the Prospect Theory.

Risk: A Matter of Perspective

Our willingness to take a risk often depends on how the situation is framed.

For example, if a doctor tells you a procedure has a 90% success rate, you might feel confident. But if instead, they mention there's a 10% failure rate, suddenly the risk seems more significant, even though the odds haven't changed.

Making Sense of Our Choices

By understanding the Prospect Theory, we gain insight into why we make certain decisions when faced with potential risks and rewards:

Safety in Certainty: We often prefer sure outcomes over uncertain ones, even if the potential reward might be higher with the gamble.

Losses Loom Large: We tend to feel the sting of losses more acutely than the pleasure of gains.

Framing Matters: How a decision is presented can drastically affect our perception of risk and reward.

Life is filled with "Fold or Call" moments. While logic and statistics play a role in our choices, our emotions and perceptions heavily influence our decisions, especially under risk. By understanding the nuances of the Prospect Theory, we can better navigate these pivotal moments, recognizing the emotional factors at play and making more informed choices.

Up next, we'll dive into how our environments and the people around us play a role in our decisions. After all, no poker game is played in isolation; every player, every bystander influences the game in their own unique way.

Chapter 7: "Hit Me": Decision Making Under Stress

Picture this: You're at a blackjack table, and the pressure is mounting. The crowd behind you is buzzing, waiting to see your next move. The dealer's eyes are on you. Do you ask for another card and risk going bust, or do you play it safe and stick? Your heart races, and suddenly, that simple decision feels monumental.

This intensity, this rush of emotions, mirrors the stress many face in their daily lives. From pressing deadlines to personal challenges, stress is a constant companion for many. But how exactly does it influence the decisions we make?

Turbulent Waters of the Mind

At its core, stress is a biological response. Think of it as your body's alarm system. It's the feeling you get when you're in choppy waters, trying to steer your ship (your mind) through a storm.

Under stress, our brain releases a flood of chemicals. These are meant to help us in the short term - they make us alert, focused, and ready to act. However, these very chemicals can cloud our judgment and influence our decisions.

Quick Decisions vs. Thoughtful Choices

When under stress, we tend to make quicker decisions. This is an evolutionary trait. If our ancestors were faced with a predator, they didn't have the luxury of mulling over their options.

But in today's world, this rapid decision-making isn't always beneficial. Think about a time you made a hasty decision under pressure and later regretted it. That's the double-edged sword of stress.

Narrowed Vision

Stress has a way of narrowing our focus. It's like having tunnel vision. Under pressure, we might zero in on immediate threats or rewards, overlooking the bigger picture.

For instance, stressed about a looming deadline, you might opt to submit a project even if it's not your best work. The immediate reward is meeting the deadline, but the long-term consequence might be a dent in your reputation for quality.

Finding Calm in the Storm

While we can't always control the stressors in our lives, we can manage how we respond:

Take a Breath: Literally. Deep breathing can help calm the mind and give you a moment of clarity.

Step Back: If possible, distance yourself from the stressful situation. Even a short break can help you see things from a fresh perspective.

Seek Counsel: Sometimes, discussing your options with someone you trust can provide valuable insights and alleviate some of the pressure.

Stress, while a natural part of life, can significantly sway our decisions. By understanding its influence, we can navigate our choices with greater awareness and intention.

In our next chapter, we'll delve into the art of decision-making in groups. Because, as you'll see, when multiple minds come together, the decision-making process takes on a whole new dynamic.

Chapter 8: "Doubling Down": Group Decision Making

Ever been in a group trying to decide where to go for dinner? One person wants sushi, another pizza, and a third can't eat gluten. The conversation goes in circles, and what started as a simple choice becomes a lively debate. This dance, this blend of voices and opinions, is the essence of group decision-making.

But why does adding more minds to a decision sometimes make it more complex? Let's dive into the dynamics of groups and see how they shape the choices we make.

The Power of Many

There's a reason we often hear the phrase "two heads are better than one." Group decisions can bring together a diverse set of perspectives, knowledge, and experiences. This rich tapestry of insights can lead to more informed and creative solutions.

For instance, a group of friends planning a trip might have someone who's great at finding deals, another who knows the best local spots, and a third who's a master scheduler. Together, they can craft an unforgettable vacation.

But Then, There's the Crowd

However, more voices can sometimes lead to a cacophony. Here's why:

Groupthink: This is when everyone starts thinking in harmony, often sidelining unique or opposing views. It's like everyone's singing the same note, and no one dares to deviate.

Social Pressure: No one likes to be the odd one out. Sometimes, people might go along with a group decision even if they have reservations, simply to fit in.

Decision Paralysis: With so many opinions on the table, groups can sometimes struggle to land on a single choice. Imagine ten people trying to pick one movie to watch - sounds daunting, right?

Finding Harmony in the Group

While group decisions can be challenging, they don't have to be chaotic. Here are some tips to keep the process smooth:

Open Floor: Encourage everyone to voice their opinions. This ensures that all perspectives are considered.

Designate a Leader: Having someone to steer the conversation can help keep discussions on track and ensure all voices are heard.

Vote: If a consensus is hard to reach, a simple majority vote can help move things forward.

Break it Down: For complex decisions, break them into smaller parts. Tackling one aspect at a time can make the process more manageable.

Whether it's a family deciding on a holiday destination or a company's boardroom meeting, group decisions are an integral part of our lives. While they bring their own set of challenges, the collective wisdom of a group can lead to decisions that a single person might never have arrived at.

As we move to our next chapter, we'll explore the fascinating realm of decisions influenced by external factors.

Chapter 9: "Cash Out": Decision Making in Business and Economics

Imagine walking into a bustling marketplace. The aroma of freshly baked goods fills the air, the sound of merchants advertising their products, and customers haggling for the best prices. It's a hive of decisions being made every second. From the baker deciding the price of his pastries to the customer choosing which stall to buy from, business and economics are all about decisions.

So, let's embark on a journey to understand the basics of how decisions are made in the vast arenas of business and economics, without getting lost in the maze of complicated terms.

Supply, Demand, and Choices

At the heart of economics is the basic principle of supply and demand. When you want to buy a fresh loaf of bread (demand), there should be a baker willing to sell it (supply). If there's only one loaf left and many want it, its price might go up. This simple dance of supply and demand drives a lot of decisions in business.

Think about the last time a popular gadget was released. Remember how everyone wanted it, and it was often sold out? That's high demand in action!

Risk and Reward: The Business Tightrope

Every businessperson, from the owner of a small coffee shop to the CEO of a multinational company, faces a common challenge: risk. Deciding to introduce a new coffee flavor or launch a new product involves weighing the potential rewards against the risks.

It's like deciding whether to jump across a stream. If you make it, you're on the other side with dry feet. If you don't, you end up with wet shoes. In business, this could mean huge profits or significant losses.

Economic Engines: Choices That Power Countries

On a larger scale, the decisions made by businesses collectively impact a country's economy. Governments also play a significant role in this. They decide on things like taxes, trade policies, and public spending. These decisions can affect everything from the price of your morning coffee to the job opportunities available in your city.

For instance, if a government decides to promote tourism, you might see more advertisements showcasing scenic spots, leading to more tourists and possibly more jobs in the tourism sector.

Staying Informed: The Key to Smart Choices

One common thread in business and economic decisions is information. The more you know, the better your decisions can be.

Market Research: This is like a business's compass. By understanding what their customers want, businesses can make products and services that are in demand.

Economic Indicators: These are the vital signs of an economy. Things like employment rates, inflation, and trade balances give policymakers an idea of the country's economic health.

The world of business and economics might seem vast and complicated, but at its core, it's all about making decisions. Decisions based on understanding supply and demand, weighing risks and rewards, and using the best information available.

Chapter 10: "Playing the Field": Cognitive Debiasing Techniques

Imagine you're playing a game of soccer. The goal is right in front of you, but instead of focusing on it, you're wearing a pair of glasses that slightly distorts everything. The goal post seems a bit off to the side, the ball appears larger than it is, and the players around seem too close or too far. This distorted view is a bit like cognitive biases: they subtly skew our perception of reality, influencing our decisions in ways we might not even notice.

But just like you'd ideally want to take off those distorting glasses to play better, in life, we can learn techniques to 'debias' our decisions. Let's explore these strategies to play the field of life with a clearer view.

Understanding the Distorted Glasses

Before we jump into the techniques, it's essential to understand what we're dealing with. Cognitive biases are like little shortcuts our brain takes. They help us process vast amounts of information quickly but sometimes lead us astray.

For example, if you've had one bad experience with a particular food, you might decide never to try it again, even if everyone else raves about it. This is a bias in action.

Strategies to Clear the View

Pause and Reflect: Before making a decision, take a moment. This brief pause can help you step back and view things more objectively. It's like wiping fog off your glasses.

Seek Other Perspectives: Remember the soccer game? Imagine having a coach on the sidelines giving you real-time feedback. Similarly, in life, getting opinions from friends, family, or colleagues can offer a fresh perspective, highlighting any biases you might have missed.

Play Devil's Advocate: Challenge your own beliefs and assumptions. By purposefully considering the opposite of what you believe, you can find gaps in your thinking or areas where bias might be influencing you.

Limit Information Overload: Just as a soccer player doesn't need to know every detail about the audience watching the match, sometimes, too much information can cloud our judgment. Focus on relevant, quality information rather than quantity.

Stay Educated: Being aware of common cognitive biases can be half the battle. If you know about them, you can be on the lookout for when they might be influencing you.

Feedback Loop: After making a decision, reflect on it. Was it the right choice? What influenced you? By analyzing your past decisions, you can get better at spotting biases in future ones.

Just as a soccer player practices to improve, understanding and working on our biases is a journey, not a destination. The goal isn't to eliminate all biases (that's nearly impossible), but to be aware of them and make more informed, clearer decisions.

In our next chapter, we'll dive into the intricate dance of emotion and logic in decision-making. Sometimes, it's not just biases that lead us astray, but the very feelings that make us human. Stay tuned!

Chapter 11: "The Winning Hand": Emotional Intelligence and Decision Making

Picture this: you're sitting at a poker table, cards in hand, chips piled in front of you. Your opponent has just raised the stakes, and everyone's eyes are on you. You can feel the tension, the excitement, the slight twinge of fear. The decision to fold or play isn't just about the cards you hold but also about reading the room, understanding your feelings, and gauging the emotions of others. This is where emotional intelligence (EI) steps into the game of decision-making.

But what is emotional intelligence, and why does it matter when we're trying to decide? Let's dive in and find out!

What's in the Cards? Emotional Intelligence Explained

At its core, emotional intelligence is the ability to recognize, understand, and manage our own emotions while also being attuned to the feelings of those around us. It's like having a superpower that lets you see and interpret the emotional currents flowing beneath the surface of human interactions.

Why is this important in decision-making? Because every choice we make isn't solely based on cold, hard facts. Our feelings, desires, and intuitions play a significant role in guiding us.

Playing it Right: The Impact of EI on Decisions

Self-awareness: Picture being at that poker table again. If you're aware of your own nervousness, you can manage it better. In life, understanding your emotions means you're less likely to make impulsive decisions based on temporary feelings.

Empathy: Just as you'd gauge an opponent's confidence or hesitation in a game, empathy helps you understand others' perspectives, leading to more compassionate and informed choices.

Emotion Regulation: Ever regretted a decision made in the heat of the moment? EI helps in keeping intense emotions in check, ensuring they don't cloud our judgment.

Enhancing Your Emotional Intelligence: Tips and Tricks

Reflection: Spend a few minutes each day reflecting on your emotions. What did you feel? Why did you feel that way? Understanding patterns in your emotions can give you better control over them.

Active Listening: When conversing with others, truly listen. This doesn't just mean hearing words, but also noticing non-verbal cues like tone, facial expressions, and body language.

Ask for Feedback: Sometimes, we might not be aware of our emotional reactions. Trusted friends or colleagues can provide insight into how we come across in various situations.

Stay Curious: When faced with a strong emotion, be it anger, joy, or frustration, get curious. Instead of reacting immediately, ask yourself what's driving that emotion.

Practice Empathy: Put yourself in others' shoes. When making decisions that impact others, try to understand their viewpoint and feelings.

The world of decisions isn't black and white. It's a spectrum of colors, driven by logic, emotion, experiences, and relationships. By honing our emotional intelligence, we can play our cards right, making decisions that are not only smart but also compassionate and holistic.

As we move into our next chapter, we'll shift our focus to the technological realm, exploring the fascinating world of algorithms and how they're shaping the decisions of the modern world. Join us as we decode the magic behind the screen!

Chapter 12: "The Final Bet": Future of Decision Making

Imagine standing on the edge of a vast, uncharted land. The horizon stretches endlessly, filled with unseen possibilities, unknown challenges, and mysteries yet to unfold. This is the frontier of our future, especially when it comes to making decisions. In a world that's evolving at breakneck speed, how we choose and the tools we use to do so are also undergoing revolutionary changes.

But instead of peering into a crystal ball, let's take a more grounded look at the factors influencing the future of decision-making in our ever-evolving world.

The Growing Landscape

Information Overload: In our digital age, we're inundated with more information than ever before. While this can be empowering, it can also be overwhelming. How do we sift through mountains of data to make informed decisions?

Technology's Hand: From AI assistants recommending our next movie to algorithms that guide crucial financial or medical decisions, technology plays a pivotal role. But remember, these tools are only as good as the hands that wield them.

Global Connections: Today, a decision made in one part of the world can ripple across continents in mere seconds, thanks to our interconnected global society. This interdependence means we have to think beyond our immediate surroundings.

Predictions for Tomorrow

Collaborative Decision Making: As challenges become more complex, decisions will be less about "me" and more about "we." Teams, communities, and even nations might need to come together to make collective choices.

Educated Intuition: With so much data available, honing our ability to quickly and accurately assess information will become an essential skill. This means blending hard facts with intuitive understanding.

Ethical Compass: As we gain more power through technology, ethical considerations will take center stage. Making the "right" decision will involve not just logic and benefits but also moral and ethical evaluations.

Charting the Course

While the terrain of the future might seem daunting, we're not without tools or maps. Here are a few strategies to navigate the evolving landscape of decision-making:

Lifelong Learning: In a world of constant change, the thirst for knowledge should never be quenched. Regularly updating our skills and understanding can help us stay ahead of the curve.

Embrace Diversity: Different perspectives enrich our decision-making process. Encouraging diversity, be it in terms of culture, gender, age, or thought, can lead to more holistic decisions.

Mindful Interactions with Technology: While technology will undoubtedly play a significant role, we must remember to use it mindfully. This means questioning algorithmic recommendations, understanding their limitations, and always using our human touch.

As we stand on the precipice of tomorrow, the choices we make will shape the world for generations to come. The journey might be filled with uncertainty, but it's also brimming with opportunity. With the right tools, mindset, and a dash of courage, we can ensure our decisions lead us to a brighter, more connected, and harmonious future.

Epilogue: "Cashing In" – Final Thoughts on the Psychology of Decision Making

Imagine you're in a grand, opulent casino. The hum of excitement is palpable as players shuffle chips and cards glide over velvety tables. You've navigated through various games, learned strategies, gauged opponents, and now, at the end of the evening, it's time to cash in your chips.

This casino is a metaphor for the journey we've been on, exploring the vast landscape of decision-making. As we come to the close, let's reflect on the power, potential, and immense value of the chips we've collected - our enhanced decision-making abilities.

The Power of Choice

Our lives are a sum of decisions, from the mundane to the monumental. Every choice carves a new path, shaping our destiny in subtle and significant ways. Recognizing the gravity of these decisions, we've delved deep into understanding the mechanics behind them, the psychological play, the biases, the interplay of emotions, and the role of the environment around us.

Empowered with this knowledge, we are better equipped, more conscious. Our decisions can become not just reactions to our surroundings, but proactive steps towards the futures we desire.

The Potential to Transform

As we've seen throughout our exploration, understanding the psychology behind decision-making isn't just about making 'better' decisions—it's about transformation. It's about personal growth, fostering healthier relationships, creating impactful communities, and even molding the very fabric of society.

Think about it. An entrepreneur with a grasp on decision-making psychology can lead a company to innovation. A teacher can inspire a generation of thinkers. A parent can nurture a child's self-confidence and worldview. The ripple effect of a single, well-informed decision can be monumental.

Mastering the Game

Understanding the psychology of decision-making isn't a one-time lesson—it's a lifelong commitment. Just as a card player continuously hones their skills, we too must be ever-vigilant, learning from our experiences, adapting to new information, and staying curious.

But why? Why is it so vital to master this art and science?

Because every decision is a declaration of who we are and what we stand for. It's an expression of our values, our beliefs, and our desires. As we continue to evolve, understanding the intricate dance of decision-making ensures that we stay true to ourselves, even as we adapt and grow.

In Conclusion

As we cash in our chips, reflecting on our journey, remember that the true value isn't in the count of the chips but in the wisdom gained. The world of decision-making is vast, intricate, and endlessly fascinating. But more than anything, it's empowering.

Thank you for joining this exploration, for challenging your perspectives, and for being open to growth. Here's to a future of enlightened choices, profound transformations, and a life richly lived. Cheers!

About Freudian Trips

Welcome to Freudian Trips, your dedicated platform for diving deep into the world of psychology. We are more than just a YouTube channel or a book publisher. We are a beacon of enlightenment, making complex psychological concepts accessible and engaging for all.

Our YouTube channel is a rich repository of psychology made simple. We take the profound and often complex ideas from the world of psychology and break them down into digestible, easy-to-understand content. From the foundational theories of Freud to the cognitive insights of Piaget, we cover a broad spectrum of psychological schools and thoughts, making psychology accessible to everyone, regardless of their background or prior knowledge.

As a book publisher, we take the same approach, transforming intricate psychological theories into comprehensible narratives. Our books are not just collections of words, but vessels of wisdom that make psychology approachable and relatable. We believe that psychology should not be confined to academic circles, but should be available to all who seek to understand the human mind and behavior.

At Freudian Trips, we believe in the power of curiosity and the pursuit of knowledge. We are here to stoke the fires of your curiosity, to guide you on your intellectual journey, and to help you navigate the fascinating world of psychology.

If you are someone who is not afraid to question, to explore, and to learn, then you are in the right place. Join us on this journey of exploration, as we make psychology easy to understand, one concept at a time.

Be sure to visit our Youtube channel at: www.freudiantrips.com/youtube

You can also visit us on the web at www.freudiantrips.com

Welcome to The Freudian Trip community. Stay curious. Stay enlightened.